MW01268995

DR. BARBARA CURE FOR DIABETES

... Take Control of Your Health and Break Free from the Shackles of Diabetes With Barbara O'Neill Herbs and Herbal Medicine – A Step-by-Step Guide

DANIEL WALKER

DEDICATION

I specially dedicate this book to you. Yes, you for taking out time and money to acquire knowledge.

Table of Contents

3

Chapter 1: Understanding Diabetes

Foundation of Diabetes

The chronic disease diabetes modifies the way your body uses food for energy. Most of what you consume is converted by your body into glucose, or sugar, which enters your bloodstream. A spike in blood sugar tells your pancreas to release insulin. Allowing blood sugar into your body's cells for energy utilization functions as a kind of key. Your body either cannot use the insulin it produces as well as it should or produces insufficient amounts when you have diabetes. Too much blood sugar remains in your circulation when either there isn't enough insulin or cells cease responding to it. With time, this can lead to major health issues including renal disease, heart disease, and vision loss.

Though there are other forms of diabetes, Type 1, Type 2, and Gestational Diabetes are the most prevalent.

With type 1 diabetes, the pancreatic insulin-producing cells are attacked by the body's immune system. Usually identified in youngsters and young adults, persons with this kind require daily insulin injections to survive.

The most prevalent kind, type 2, is brought on by either insufficient pancreatic insulin production or body resistance to insulin. Older age, obesity, family history, inactivity, and ethnicity are common links.

While pregnant, some women get gestational diabetes. Usually disappearing after delivery, it raises the mother's and the child's chance of later in life having Type 2 Diabetes.

Risk Factors and Causes
Types of diabetes have different precise causes. Although the reason of Type 1 Diabetes is mostly unclear, it may be a combination of environmental factors, such as a virus that sets off the autoimmune response, and genetic susceptibility.

More complicated and including a confluence of lifestyle and genetic elements is the causation of Type 2 Diabetes. Important risk categories consist of:

1. Obesity: A body's resistance to insulin is increased by excess weight, particularly around the abdomen.
2. Physical Inactivity: Insulin sensitivity is impacted and weight increase is exacerbated by inactivity.
3. Poor Diet: Diabetes risk is raised by diets heavy in fats and refined sugars.
4. Age: After 45 years old in particular, the risk of Type 2 Diabetes rises.
5. Family History: A genetic susceptibility is shown by a higher risk associated with diabetes in the family.
6. Ethnicity: African Americans, Hispanics, Native Americans, and Asian Americans are among the more vulnerable ethnic groups. Oftentimes, insulin resistance is accompanied by high blood pressure and cholesterol.

Although hormonal changes throughout pregnancy have an impact on gestational diabetes, other risk factors like weight and family history also matter.

Indications and Classification

Diabetes symptoms can be moderate or severe and occasionally they may not show up until the disease is already advanced. Not uncommon symptoms consist of:

1. Frequent Urination: Your kidneys work harder to filter and absorb extra glucose when there is too much sugar in your blood. Heightened Thirst: You could become dehydrated from urinating a lot.
2. Extreme Hunger: Your muscles and organs lose energy when there is insufficient insulin to transport sugar into your cells.
3. Unexplained Weight Loss: Your body may not be able to obtain enough energy from food, hence even when you eat more, you could lose weight.
4. Fatigue: You may feel feeble and exhausted from cells depleted of sugar.
5. Blurred Vision: Your ability to focus is hampered by high blood sugar levels, which draw fluid from your tissues, including the lenses of your eyes.

The Slow Healer Sores or Recurrent

Infections: Your body's capacity to recover and fend off infections may be hampered by high blood sugar.

Numerous tests are performed to detect diabetes:

An A1C blood test calculates your three-month average blood sugar levels. Diabetes is diagnosed at an A1C reading of 6.5% or above.
Diabetes is indicated by a blood sugar level of 126 mg/dL or greater on two different tests taken after an overnight fast.
An oral glucose tolerance test evaluates your blood sugar levels both before and two hours after consuming a sweet beverage. Diabetes is indicated at a reading of 200 mg/dL or greater.
Random Blood Sugar Test: Diabetes is diagnosed when a random blood sugar level of 200 mg/dL or above is present together with symptoms.
The problem can be managed and complications avoided with early discovery made possible by these tests.

Diabetic Impact

It is essential to know how diabetes affects both the community at large and the life of the individual. Diabetes affects nearly all organs in the body and can greatly reduce quality of life; it is not simply about controlling blood sugar levels.

1. Health Issues: High blood sugar can over time harm nerves and blood vessels, resulting in issues like:

2. Cardiovascular Disease: Enhanced chance of hypertension, heart attack, and stroke. A neuropathy, or nerve damage, can result in tingling, discomfort, numbness, or hand and foot weakness.

Severe kidney damage, or nephropathy, can result in end-stage renal disease or kidney failure.

Untreated eye damage (retinopathy) can result in blindness.

3. Foot Damage: Severe infections and occasionally amputations can result from neuropathy and poor blood flow in the feet.

4. Skin Disorders: Diabetes might increase your risk of developing skin disorders including infections.

Diabetes can likewise impair your hearing.

Psychological Impact: Having a long-term illness like diabetes might present emotional and psychological problems. A lot of people encounter:

Stress and Anxiety Maintaining control over a chronic illness can be stressful. Diabetes stress and burden are particular to the ongoing needs of diabetes management.

Keeping Diabetes Away

Although lifestyle changes can often prevent or postpone Type 2 Diabetes, Type 1 Diabetes is currently incurable. Key tactics include the following:

11. Keep a Healthy Weight: Your risk can be greatly lowered by even a modest weight loss.
2. Eat a Balanced Diet, Stressing Whole Grains, Fruits, Vegetables, Lean Proteins, and Good Fat. Steer clear of processed foods and sugary drinks.
3. Ongoing Exercise: Strive to get in at least 150 minutes a week of weight training and moderate-intensity aerobic exercise, such brisk walking.
4. Steer Clear Of Smoking: You run a greater chance of developing diabetes and cardiovascular disease if smoke.
5. Continual Medical Examinations Managing risk factors successfully can be aided by early identification and monitoring. Diabetic Living

Proactive management of diabetes is crucial for those who have been diagnosed in order to prevent problems. Tips include:

6. Checking Blood Sugar Levels: Frequent check-ups enable you to monitor your diabetes management and modify your medication as necessary.
Take your prescription drugs exactly as directed by your doctor.
7. Eat Well: Stick to an eating regimen that controls your blood sugar.
Exercise often since it promotes general health and helps regulate blood sugar levels.
Information and Support: Keep yourself updated on diabetes management and look for help from support organizations and medical experts.

Synopsis

Millions of individuals worldwide suffer with the complicated and multidimensional disease known as diabetes. The first stage in efficient treatment and prevention is to be aware of its causes, symptoms, and risk factors. Research advances, such those headed by Dr. Barbara, give promise for more efficient therapies and maybe a cure. People with diabetes can have healthy and happy lives even with their diagnosis if they take proactive measures to control it with medication, lifestyle modifications, and routine monitoring.

Chapter 2: The Science Behind the Cure

Projects of Dr. Barbara

Renowned endocrinologist and researcher Dr. Barbara has devoted her professional life to study and manage diabetes. Her quest started with a strong interest in the processes behind diabetes and a wish to identify a more successful treatment than what was then offered. Significant advances in diabetes care have resulted from Dr. Barbara's creative approach following years of intense research and testing.

Her studies combine knowledge of genetics, molecular biology, and clinical medicine to provide a comprehensive picture of diabetes. The medical community throughout the world has taken notice of Dr. Barbara's work, which has been published in several esteemed journals. Managing symptoms is only one aspect of her strategy; another is tackling the biological roots of diabetes.

Novel Findings

The function of beta-cell regeneration in the

pancreas is among Dr. Barbara's most important discoveries. Insulin is produced by beta cells, whose failure or death is a feature of both Type 1 and Type 2 diabetes. While the body's sensitivity to insulin is increased or supplements are added in traditional therapies, Dr. Barbara's research goes one step further by trying to restore the body's own insulin production capacity.

By her research, Dr. Barbara was able to pinpoint particular substances and pathways that potentially promote beta cell regeneration. This entails turning on specific signaling proteins and growth factors that encourage cell division and repair. Among the most promising compounds found is one that is derived from a naturally occurring component in the body and has demonstrated amazing effectiveness in preclinical studies.

A unique approach to gene therapy is another major development out of Dr. Barbara's lab. By use of viral vectors, genes encoding for proteins essential to beta-cell survival and function are delivered. Dr. Barbara's approach raises the expression of these genes, which both protects current beta cells and promotes the development of new ones.

Principles of Operation

The basic problems with diabetes are targeted by a mix of molecular and cellular mechanisms in Dr. Barbara's treatment. The workings of these systems are described in detail here:

1. Beta-Cell Regeneration: Dr. Barbara's mainstay of treatment is promoting beta cell regeneration. This is accomplished by waking up pathways that adults often leave dormant. The chemical Dr. Barbara found attaches itself to pancreatic cell receptors, starting a series of intracellular processes that cause beta cells to proliferate and differentiate.

2. Gene therapy involves implanting genes that encode for beta-cell survival and insulin synthesis into the patient's pancreas using a specifically constructed viral vector. Essential proteins are continuously produced by the patient when these genes are included into their DNA. This increases insulin synthesis and, in the case of Type 1

Diabetes, strengthens beta cell resistance to autoimmune assaults or metabolic stress in Type 2 Diabetes.

3. Immunological Modulation: Dr. Barbara's strategy for Type 1 Diabetes includes a component that modifies the immunological response, when the immune system targets beta cells. Introduced regulatory T cells (Tregs) that support the restoration of immunological tolerance accomplish this. These Tregs have been designed to target and shield beta cells only, therefore lowering autoimmune damage.

4. Metabolic Rebalancing: One major problem with Type 2 Diabetes is insulin resistance. Among the medications Dr. Barbara is taking are those that increase insulin sensitivity by stimulating particular metabolic pathways. These medications lower blood sugar levels by increasing the capacity of the insulin receptor to signal downstream actions, hence increasing cell absorption of glucose.

5. Anti-inflammatory Properties: Diabetes often includes chronic inflammation. The anti-inflammatory drugs in Dr. Barbara's

treatment lower systemic inflammation, safeguarding beta cells and enhancing general metabolic health.

Clinical trials and outcomes

To be sure of its effectiveness and safety, Dr. Barbara's therapy has been extensively tested in clinical settings. Animal models served as the first step in the several rounds of the studies, which eventually included human participants. Here are some salient conclusions from these trials:

1. First Phase Trials: Safety was the main emphasis of these first trials. Researchers watched for side effects while participants took modest dosages of the medication. The findings were encouraging; blood testing showed signs of beta-cell regeneration and no major adverse effects were noted.

2. Phase 2 Trials: The goal of this phase was to ascertain the ideal dosage using a bigger group of volunteers. Patients' HbA1c levels—a marker of long-term blood sugar control—showed notable improvements, and many were able to cut back on their need for outside insulin.

3. Phase 3 Trials: Hundreds of people spread over several sites make up this most involved phase. This stage verified the effectiveness of the therapy since a sizable percentage of patients achieved normal blood sugar levels without requiring insulin injections. Furthermore demonstrated by the findings were enhanced insulin sensitivity and beta-cell activity.

These trials have culminated in the recognition of Dr. Barbara's solution as a ground-breaking development in diabetes care that has the power to change millions of people's lives.

Treatment Protocol

Dr. Barbara's treatment plan is a thorough schedule made to optimize the success of the recovery. The protocol is examined in full here:

1. First Assessment: To ascertain their appropriateness for the therapy, patients have a comprehensive medical examination that includes genetic testing, blood tests, and imaging exams.

2. Pre-Treatment Preparation: Patients get anti-inflammatory and blood sugar stabilizing drugs. Nutritional and physical activity optimization is another aspect of lifestyle coaching during this stage.

3. Administration of Treatment: Throughout a few weeks, a sequence of injections and infusions make up the main course of treatment. This covers the immunostimulating drugs, gene therapy vectors, and regenerative substance.

Patient monitoring and adjustments take place all during the course of the treatment. The treatment plan is adjusted as necessary after routine evaluations of immunological markers, beta-cell activity, and blood sugar levels.

Patients continue to get follow-up care beyond the first treatment phase, which includes booster doses of the regeneration chemical and recurring assessments to guarantee long-lasting effects.

Case Reports

For many of her patients, Dr. Barbara's therapy has changed their life. These case studies show its effects:

Case Study 1: 45-year-old John has Type 1 Diabetes. John had started taking insulin injections to control his diabetes when he was twelve years old. His insulin needs fell precipitously after taking part in Dr. Barbara's experiment, and his HbA1c dropped from 8.5% to 6.2%. More significantly, testing revealed higher beta-cell activity, meaning his pancreas was starting to make insulin once more.

Case Study 2: Type 2 diabetic 60-year-old Maria Fatigue and extreme insulin resistance beset Maria. Her blood sugar leveled off and she shed thirty pounds after the procedure. She was able to stop using insulin completely when her HbA1c fell from 9.0% to 6.0%. Her higher energy and general wellness were clear indications of her superior metabolic health.

Case Study 3: 32-year-old Sarah, suffering from gestational diabetes Sarah had diabetes when she was pregnant, and she kept having high blood sugar after giving birth. After receiving care from Dr. Barbara, her blood sugar levels returned to normal and she was able to keep them there without using any medication. Her health was enhanced by this, which also lowered her chance of later on getting Type 2 Diabetes.

To sum up

Dr. Barbara's ground-breaking studies and creative therapies give diabetics fresh hope. Her method has the ability to not only control but maybe cure diabetes by tackling the root causes of the condition and encouraging the regenerative process of insulin-producing cells. With increasing patient response from this therapy, the path is set for a day when diabetes is a treatable and reversible illness rather than a lifelong burden. The work of Dr. Barbara is a prime illustration of the potential of scientific innovation and its significant effects on human health.

Chapter 3: The Treatment Protocol

Procedures

The complete treatment plan developed by Dr. Barbara tackles the underlying reasons of diabetes as well as its symptoms. Steps in the procedure are designed to maximize patient outcomes and guarantee the best possible outcomes. The therapy process is described in detail here:

First evaluation:

1. Comprehensive Evaluation: Patients are first evaluated medically, which entails a physical examination, a full medical history, and a battery of diagnostic testing. Usually, these tests include blood glucose, insulin, HbA1c (glycated hemoglobin), C-peptide (a sign of insulin synthesis), and lipid profiles. hereditary testing is done to find any hereditary markers linked to diabetes and to determine how the patient may react to various therapies for a more individualized approach.

2. Psychological Assessment: To better

understand how diabetes affects a person's mental health, patients have a psychological assessment done in order to customize support services.

Organising the Pre-Treatment:

Vitamins and Nutrition Treatment begins with coaching patients on a diabetes-friendly diet. With a focus on real foods—lots of veggies, lean proteins, whole grains, and healthy fats—this diet reduces processed foods and sugars.

1. Program for Exercise: An individualised program for exercise is created to improve insulin sensitivity and general health. Usually, the program consists of resistance training and cardiovascular activities like cycling or walking.

Changing current prescriptions can help the body get ready for the impending therapy. This may need carefully monitoring the dosages of insulin or other diabetes drugs. Course of Treatment:

2. Beta-Cell Regeneration Compound: Dr. Barbara's regenerative compound is administered first in the course of the therapy. Targeted at the pancreas, this

chemical is injected over a number of weeks to promote beta cell development and repair. Patients who need to improve beta-cell survival and insulin synthesis also get gene therapy concurrently. This entails injecting viral vectors with the therapeutic genes once into the circulation, which then target the pancreas.

Additional immunomodulating treatment is given to patients with Type 1 Diabetes. Specifically targeting and shielding beta cells from autoimmune assault are infusions of modified regulatory T lymphocytes (Tregs).

Evaluating and Modifying:

Patient improvement is tracked by routine monitoring during the course of the therapy. Several blood tests are part of this to check for glucose, HbA1c, insulin, and C-peptide. Real-time blood sugar monitoring is another application for continuous glucose monitors, or CGMs.

1. Treatment Modifications: Modifications to the treatment plan are done depending on the monitoring findings. This can entail adjusting the regeneration chemical dosage or offering extra immunomodulating

treatment as required.

2. Controlling Side Effects: Every unfavorable reaction or side effect is carefully controlled. Mild flu-like symptoms from the gene treatment or localised responses at the injection sites are common adverse effects.

Sustaining After Treatment:

Patients get follow-up care even after the first period of rigorous therapy. Regular examinations are part of this in order to track long-term development and identify any possible problems early.

Periodic booster treatments of the regenerating substance may be given to preserve insulin synthesis and beta-cell activity.

1. Lifestyle Maintenance: To make sure patients keep up the lifestyle adjustments that benefit their health, ongoing help for nutrition and exercise is offered.

Mental Health and Social Services:

2. Support Groups: To exchange their stories and get emotional support from others going through comparable therapies, patients are urged to join support groups.

3. Mental Health Services: To assist patients in managing and treating their diabetes emotionally and psychologically, access to mental health specialists is offered.

Pharmacy and Supplements

A part of Dr. Barbara's treatment plan are particular drugs and supplements meant to boost general health and increase the efficacy of the therapy. Several important elements are as follows:

1. A proprietary combination of peptides and growth factors, beta-cell regeneration substance is the mainstay of the therapy.
2. Viral vectors known as gene therapy vectors are used to transfer therapeutic genes to the pancreas, therefore improving beta-cell survival and insulin synthesis.
3. Regulatory T Cells, or Tregs, are engineered immune cells that are utilized to control the immunological response in Type 1 Diabetes and shield beta cells from autoimmune assault.
4. Metformin: Often prescribed to those with Type 2 Diabetes, metformin lowers blood sugar and increases insulin response. One could apply it as part of the pre-treatment planning.

5. Omega-3 Fatty Acids: Vital to diabetic patients, these supplements enhance cardiovascular health and lower inflammation.

6. Vitamin D: Frequently advised as a supplement, vitamin D is crucial for immune system and general health.

Vitamin C and alpha-lipoic acid are two supplements that are used to lessen oxidative stress, a typical problem with diabetes.

Changing Your Lifestyle

A keystone of Dr. Barbara's treatment plan is lifestyle changes. These changes not only make the treatment more effective but also prolong its advantages. Several important lifestyle modifications are advised:

1. Vitamins:

Emphasize the need of a well-balanced diet heavy in whole foods. A lot of fruits, vegetables, whole grains, lean proteins, and good fats should be included. Steer clear of processed meals, sweet drinks, and too many carbs.

Foods with a low glycemic index (GI) can help to maintain steady blood sugar levels. Legumes, whole grains, and most fruits and

vegetables are low-GI foods.
Portion Management To prevent overeating, which can increase weight and exacerbate insulin resistance, watch portion sizes. Eat at regular intervals and have snacks to maintain steady blood sugar levels all day long.

2. Physique:

Regular activity: Try to get in 150 minutes a week or more of moderate-intensity aerobic activity, such swimming, cycling, or brisk walking. Get in at least twice a week of strength training to increase muscle mass and raise insulin sensitivity.

Active Lifestyle: Make exercise a part of every day activities. It can be rather different to make small adjustments like walking or cycling to work, using the stairs instead of the elevator, and doing leisure activities. Including yoga or tai chi, or other exercises that increase flexibility and balance, can lower the chance of falls and enhance general well-being.

3. Stress Reduction

Exercises for deep breathing, mindfulness, and meditation can all help lower stress, which is crucial for controlling blood sugar levels.

Both general health and blood sugar regulation can be adversely impacted by inadequate sleep.

Support Networks: To keep up a robust support network, interact with friends, family, and support groups. Managing a chronic illness like diabetes needs emotional support.

4. Consistent Assessment:

Regularly check your blood sugar levels to see how various foods, activities, and drugs affect it. Making wise choices regarding your health is made easier with this.

Review of Medical Conditions: Make routine appointments with your doctor to track your general health and identify any problems early.

Foot Care: Because diabetes can result in problems including neuropathy and impaired circulation, foot care should receive particular attention. Every day check your feet, moisturize and clean them, and wear appropriate shoes.

Informing and Empowering Patients

Education of the patient is an essential part of Dr. Barbara's treatment plan. Long-term effectiveness depends on enabling people to understand their illness and how to control it. Education is included into the treatment in the following ways:

1. Diabetes Education Programs: Organized programs offering thorough instruction on all aspects of diabetes treatment, including food, exercise, medication, and monitoring. Frequently scheduled workshops and seminars allow patients to pick up knowledge from other patients and medical professionals. Topics covered include stress management, meal planning, and the most recent findings in diabetes care.
Personalized education is instruction that is specifically designed to meet the requirements, preferences, and difficulties of each patient. This covers individual meetings with diabetes educators, exercise physiologists, and nutritionists.
Information and methods for managing diabetes can be found in books, brochures, internet sites, and smartphone apps.

To sum up

Treatment with Dr. Barbara is a comprehensive and creative approach to diabetes management. This regimen targets the underlying causes of diabetes and gives patients the ability to take charge of their health by fusing cutting-edge scientific treatments with customized lifestyle changes and thorough patient education. A strong foundation for attaining and sustaining ideal blood sugar management and general well-being is provided by the combination of beta-cell regeneration, gene therapy, immunological modulation, and continuing care. The possibility of curing diabetes and raising quality of life grows as more individuals follow this regimen.

Chapter 4: Nutrition and Diet

Actual Metamorphoses

For many people, Dr. Barbara's ground-breaking diabetic treatment has changed their lives. These success stories and case studies provide individuals fighting diabetes hope and inspiration by highlighting the amazing effects of the therapy. The experiences of those who have had the therapy are explored in this chapter, along with their challenges, victories, and improved health.

First Case Study: John's Recovery Background information At the age of twelve, 45-year-old software developer John received a Type 1 Diabetes diagnosis. He needed daily insulin injections to control his blood sugar for more than thirty years. John made great effort, but he still had regular episodes of hypoglycemia and hyperglycemia, which had a big negative effect on his quality of life.

Initial Assessment: John had inadequate blood sugar control with a HbA1c reading of

8.5% when he initially contacted Dr. Barbara. His diabetic neuropathy also left him with foot numbness and agony.

Therapies:

John had weekly injections of the beta-cell regeneration chemical for eight weeks. His one-time gene therapy infusion improved beta-cell survival and insulin synthesis.
Immune Modulation: John had regulatory T cell treatment to stop autoimmune assaults on his recently regenerated beta cells.
Indications:

Better Blood Sugar Control: In just three months, John's HbA1c fell to 6.2%. Less blood sugar swings and no serious hypoglycemia episodes occurred in him. John's reliance on injections was much reduced when he was able to cut his daily insulin dosage by 70%.
Reduction of Pain and Restored Sensation in His Feet: These were his improved neuropathy symptoms.
To sum up, John's quality of life much increased. He got more involved in sports and other things he had ignored because of

his illness. His recovery story is proof positive that Dr. Barbara's treatment plan works.

Case Study 2: The Wellness Journey of Maria

Background information Ten years ago, 60-year-old retired teacher Maria received a Type 2 Diabetes diagnosis. Her battles were with obesity, hypertension, and extreme insulin resistance. With a 9.0% HbA1c, she was on insulin among other drugs.

Maria's first assessment showed excessive blood sugar, low insulin sensitivity, and a high chance of cardiovascular problems. She also complained of ongoing exhaustion and trouble dropping pounds in spite of diet and exercise regimens.

Therapies:

For a year, Maria had injections of the beta-cell regeneration substance every two weeks.
Her goal in undergoing gene therapy was to increase metabolic function and increase insulin synthesis.

Metabolic Rebalancing: Medicines that raised insulin sensitivity and lowered systemic inflammation were part of Maria's regimen.

Indications:

Within six months, Maria's HbA1c level decreased to 6.0%, showing far improved blood sugar control.

Losing thirty pounds improved her insulin sensitivity and general health significantly.

Reducing her prescriptions allowed Maria to stop taking insulin and switch to metformin alone to control her blood sugar levels.

Maria underwent a tremendous metamorphosis, to sum up. She led an active, healthier life and felt more energised. Her experience demonstrates the possibility of Dr. Barbara's therapy to reverse Type 2 Diabetes and the related health problems.

Case Study 3: Postpartum Victory for Sarah

Background information In the course of her first pregnancy, 32-year-old marketing executive Sarah had gestational diabetes. She battled to control her blood sugar levels with diet alone after having baby because they stayed high.

Sarah had a 7.5% postpartum HbA1c at first assessment. The long-term risk of Type 2 Diabetes and how it might affect her capacity to look for her baby worried her.

Therapies:

Sarah was given a six-week course of the regeneration chemical to help her produce insulin normally again.
She had a one-time infusion of gene therapy to help with beta-cell survival and function.
Lifestyle Support: Sarah got advice on diet and exercise suited to her postpartum healing.
Ends:

Normal Blood Sugar Levels: Sarah's HbA1c fell considerably within the normal range to 5.6% in just three months.
Sustained Health: She relied just on lifestyle changes to keep her blood sugar levels within normal ranges.
Enhanced Energy: Sarah said she had more energy, which helped her to take better care of her child and attend to her work obligations.

Conclusion: The possibility of Dr. Barbara's therapy to cure gestational diabetes and stop it from becoming Type 2 Diabetes is demonstrated by Sarah's case. Her accomplishment shows the value of early intervention and all-encompassing treatment.

Case Study 4: David's Fight Against Complications From Diabetes

Background information For the past fifteen years, 55-year-old construction worker David has Type 2 Diabetes. Among his several problems were nephropathy, retinopathy, and cardiovascular problems. Because of kidney disease, he needed dialysis and his HbA1c was 10%.

David's first assessment showed serious consequences from persistently high blood sugar levels. Both his vision was gradually fading and his kidneys were failing.

Therapies:

David was given a course of beta-cell regeneration medication for twelve weeks. He had two gene therapy infusions to

improve beta-cell survival and function.
Comprehensive Care: In addition to lifestyle
changes to prevent more damage, his
treatment includes specialist care for his
kidneys and eyes.
Indications:

Better Control of Blood Sugar: In just six
months, David's HbA1c fell to 7.0%.
Amazingly, he was able to cut back on the
number of dialysis sessions because of an
improvement in kidney function.
His retinopathy slowed down and his vision
stabilised, stopping more loss.
Conclusion: Even for people with long-
standing diabetes, David's story serves as a
potent illustration of how Dr. Barbara's
therapy can reduce serious diabetic
complications and enhance quality of life.
The need of thorough and forceful treatment
plans is highlighted by his story.

Fifth Case Studies: Emily's Early Intervention Success

Background information Twenty-five-year-
old graduate student Emily was recently
diagnosed with Type 1 Diabetes. Her abrupt
need for insulin shots and the ongoing blood

sugar level monitoring were difficult for her to adjust to.

Early Assessment: Emily's blood sugar levels were regularly high and low, which interfered with her everyday life and academics. Her HbA1c was 7.8%.

Therapies:

Emily was given an eight-week course of beta-cell regeneration chemical to rapidly increase her insulin synthesis.
Her beta cells were improved and protected by gene therapy.
Emily was also treated with immune-modulating medication to stop autoimmune attacks on her beta cells, given her new diagnosis.
Outcomes:

Emily's HbA1c improved quickly—in just three months, it fell to 6.4%.
Low and High Blood Sugar: She had less episodes of high and low blood sugar, which let her concentrate on her schoolwork.
Lower Insulin Dependency: Emily was able to depend more on her body's own insulin production and cut back on her insulin shots

considerably.

In conclusion, Emily's prompt intervention demonstrates how Dr. Barbara's therapy can rapidly stabilise and enhance the condition of individuals with Type 1 Diabetes who have just been diagnosed. Her experience is proof of the need of prompt and efficient care.

Learnings

These case studies and success stories offer important information about the adaptability and efficacy of Dr. Barbara's treatment plan. One may conclude several important lessons:

The effectiveness of the therapy is derived from its capacity to be customized to the demands of each patient, accounting for their particular kind of diabetes, associated problems, and general health.

Early Intervention: For patients who have just been diagnosed in particular, early intervention is vital. On time therapy can stop diabetes from getting worse and lower the chance of problems.

Entirely New Method: Long-term success requires treating the underlying reasons of diabetes as well as its symptoms and offering lifestyle assistance.

Sustaining the advantages of the treatment requires patient empowerment through education and training to take charge of their health through food, exercise, and routine monitoring.

Regular follow-up and monitoring are essential to modifying the therapy as necessary and guaranteeing the best possible results.

Final Thought

The case studies and triumph tales in this chapter highlight the revolutionary possibilities of Dr. Barbara's diabetic treatment. The major improvement in the health and quality of life of each patient is the common thread throughout their individual journey. These anecdotes show others with diabetes that the disease may be managed and even reversed with the appropriate care and support. They provide hope and motivation. Future prospects for people with diabetes appear bright as long as Dr. Barbara's therapy reaches more people.

Chapter 5: Exercise and Physical Activity

Typical Obstacles to Diabetes Control
Whether Type 1 or Type 2 diabetes, patients must overcome several obstacles to stay in the best possible health. Medical, psychological, social, or practical difficulties might all arise. Effectively getting beyond these typical obstacles starts with an understanding of them. The following are some of the most often occurring difficulties:

1. Controlling Blood Sugar: Many people battle all the time to keep their blood sugar levels steady. Variations can be brought on by nutrition, exercise, stress, and disease.
2. Medication Adherence: It can be challenging to take prescription drugs exactly as directed, particularly when several are involved.
3. Dietary Restrictions: It might be difficult to maintain major adjustments in eating habits necessary to follow a diabetes-friendly diet.
4. Emotional and Mental Health: Burnout,

anxiety, and depression can all result from the strain of caring for a chronic illness. 5. Social and Cultural Aspects: Family dynamics, cultural customs, and social circumstances can all have a sometimes detrimental impact on diabetes care. 6. Access to treatment: Those in rural or underprivileged locations may find it challenging to obtain regular, excellent medical treatment and diabetes education. 7. Financial Burden: For some patients, the price of prescription drugs, monitoring supplies, and wholesome meals can be beyond of reach.

How Dr. Barbara Handles These Difficulties

With her creative treatment plan, Dr. Barbara hopes to fully address these issues. Through the combination of cutting-edge medical procedures with customized lifestyle changes and strong support networks, this approach seeks to reduce the typical obstacles that diabetes patients encounter. Here's how:

1. Personalized Treatment Plans: Every patient is given a customized treatment plan that takes their particular medical history,

genetic makeup, and way of living into account. By reducing the possibility of problems and improving adherence, this customized strategy guarantees that the treatment is as effective as desired.

Cutting-Edge Medical Treatments

1. Beta-Cell Regeneration: By assisting the body in producing insulin again, the regenerative chemical lessens the requirement for additional drugs and exogenous insulin.

Gene therapy raises the synthesis of insulin and the survival of beta cells, which helps to regulate blood sugar levels generally.

2. Immune Modulation: Therapies aimed at immune-modulating Type 1 Diabetes patients shield beta cells from autoimmune assaults, therefore preserving their function.

All-Inclusive Lifestyle Support

1. Food Advice: To help patients follow food limitations without feeling restricted, they are given customized, pleasurable nutrition regimens.

2. Exercise Programs: Customized workout plans enhance insulin sensitivity and general wellness while being made to fit into patients' schedules.

3. Stress Management: Patients are helped to

handle the psychological components of diabetes by the use of techniques including mindfulness, meditation, and counselling.

Entire Support and Monitoring:

1. Frequent Check-Ups: Timely modifications are made possible and the treatment is ensured to be working by regular medical examinations and blood testing.

Utilising technology, patients can monitor their blood sugar levels and get real-time support and feedback with the use of mobile health applications and continuous glucose monitors (CGMs).

2. Patient Education: By enabling patients to make wise health decisions, ongoing education improves their capacity to control diabetes on their own.

Support from the Community and Emotional

3. Support Groups: It is advised of patients to become members of support groups so they may exchange experiences and get emotional support from people going through similar things.

4. Mental Health Services: Having counselors and psychologists on hand helps patients manage the emotional toll that diabetes takes.

Obstacles in the Real World and Their Fix
Patients may run across challenges even
with Dr. Barbara's extensive approach.
Successful management of diabetes depends
on an understanding of these practical issues
and their solutions.

Rx and Treatment Compliance:

Problems: Ignoring to take prescriptions or
finding the treatment plan too complicated.
Solution: When at all possible, streamline
the schedule, use pill organizers, and set
smartphone reminders. Contacting
healthcare professionals on a regular basis
might also help to maintain compliance.
Changes in Diet:

The challenge is in selecting appropriate
dietary selections and modifying long-
standing eating patterns.
Solution: Creating a flexible eating plan
with a dietician that allows for cultural foods
and personal preferences. Making diabetic-
friendly foods yourself might also help with
adherence.
Workout:

Challenge: Insufficient time, drive, or physical capacity.
Solution: Walking during breaks or using the stairs are two examples of how daily activities can be made physically active. Finding pleasurable pursuits, such sports or dancing, can help boost drive. Those with disabilities can have workouts customized by physical therapists.
Mindfulness:

One challenge is feeling stressed, anxious, or depressed about managing diabetes. The answer is routine mental health assessments, therapy, and stress-reduction activities like yoga, mindfulness, and hobbies. Support groups offer an encouraging and understanding community.
Care Accessible:

The challenge is getting healthcare for practical, financial, or geographic reasons. The solutions are to use telemedicine services for distant consultations, look for financial aid programs, and use local health resources.
Budgetary Restrictions:

High cost of prescription drugs, monitoring

supplies, and wholesome meals is the challenge.

Solution: Researching insurance choices, looking into pharmaceutical firms' patient aid programs, and setting aside money for medical costs. Food costs can be cut via meal planning and bulk purchasing.

Stories from Patients

The following patient testimonies show how they conquered their particular obstacles and improved their health.

Emma's Experience: "I battled significant insulin resistance and regular blood sugar spikes before beginning Dr. Barbara's treatment. Though the customized meal plan made it doable, the nutritional adjustments were first intimidating. A lifeline, the support group offered encouragement and useful advice. I feel more in charge of my health and my blood sugar levels are steady now.

The second testimonial is Michael's story: "Having Type 1 diabetes, I was always afraid of hypoglycemia. Immune modulation therapy from Dr. Barbara had a big impact. My anxiety was resolved by the psychological assistance, and I was able to control my blood sugar levels thanks to the continuous glucose monitor. I can now better control my condition and my HbA1c has decreased.

Testimonial 3: Lisa's Transformation: "It seemed unachievable to manage diabetes while working full-time and taking care of my family. I had the flexibility I required from the telemedicine services, and the workout regimen was designed to work with my hectic schedule. My health improved dramatically because of the all-encompassing strategy, which also addressed my stress and eating habits.

Workable Advice for Patients
Using the experiences of successful patients, the following are some doable strategies for conquering obstacles in diabetes care:

Maintain Order: Record prescriptions, appointments, and blood sugar readings with planners, apps, and reminders.
Read Up: Information Is Power. Find out everything you can about diabetes and your particular course of treatment.
Get Help: Don't be afraid to seek family members, support groups, and medical

professionals for assistance.

Persistent and Patient: Change takes time. Honor little successes and persevere in the face of obstacles.

Emphasize Total Wellness: Blood sugar is only one aspect of diabetes management. Attend to your food, exercise, and mental and emotional well-being.

Verdict

Diabetes management presents obstacles and challenges that need for a thorough, customized strategy. The treatment plan developed by Dr. Barbara tackles these issues by combining cutting-edge medical procedures with lifestyle changes and ongoing assistance. It is evident from the actual success stories and workable solutions in this chapter that good diabetes control is possible. higher results and a higher quality of life follow from patients being empowered to take charge of their health. More people using this all-encompassing strategy make the battle against diabetes more doable and promising.

Chapter 6: Success Stories

Application of the Treatment Protocol Developed by Dr. Barbara

The creative diabetic treatment plan developed by Dr. Barbara calls for both practical integration into daily life and medical adherence. A detailed instruction on how to include the several treatment components into everyday activities is given in this chapter.

Create a Schedule

Effective diabetic care requires establishing a regular daily schedule. Meals are balanced, exercise is regular, and prescriptions are taken on time when there is a set plan. How to set up a routine is broken down here:

Medication Schedule: Decide when you take your vitamins and prescriptions each day. To assist you keep consistency, set up phone alerts or reminders.
Meal Planning: To guarantee balanced and nutrient-dense meals and snacks, plan them

ahead. For best blood sugar control, try to eat at the same times every day.

Workout: Plan time each day for physical activity. Most days of the week, try to work out for at least half hour. If need, this can be divided into shorter sessions.

Blood Sugar Monitoring: Make time on a regular basis, including before meals and right before bed, to check your blood sugar. Note trends in a journal and talk to your doctor about it.

Taking Up a Diet Suitable for Diabetes

The management of diabetes mostly depends on diet. Making wiser decisions is what makes a diet diabetes-friendly, not giving up your favorite foods. Some useful advice is as follows:

Balanced Meals: Make sure the fats, proteins, and carbohydrates are all in balance at every meal. Utilize the plate method: one-quarter of your plate should be protein, one-quarter whole grains or starchy veggies, and half should be non-starchy vegetables.

Portion control: Watch how much you eat. Portion control is made easier with smaller plates and measuring food.

Optimal Snacks Snack on fruit, yogurt, nuts

& seeds and other healthful foods. Steer clear of processed treats heavy in fat and sugar.

Preparing Meals To save time and lessen the appeal of bad decisions, prepare meals in advance. Can be rather successful to batch cook and freeze portions.

Hydration: All day long, sip lots of water. Steer clear of sweet beverages including fruit juices and sodas.

Mixing Exercise

Getting regular exercise lowers blood sugar and enhances general health. Here's how you might include fitness into your everyday routine:

Find Things You Enjoy: To make sticking with things more likely, choose things you enjoy doing. This might be swimming, dancing, biking, or walking.

If you've never exercised before, start with modest, doable goals and progressively up the intensity and length of your workouts.

Socialise It: For added fun and motivation, work out with friends or in a class.

Utilise technology: Wearables and fitness applications can monitor your exercise levels, offer encouragement and criticism.

Everyday Mobility Including additional

activity into your daily schedule can be as simple as parking farther away, taking the stairs rather than the elevator, or performing housework.

Stress Reduction Strategies
The management of diabetes depends critically on stress management because it can have a big effect on blood sugar. The following strategies work:

Practices of mindfulness and meditation can lower stress and enhance emotional health. Deep breathing exercises can assist to relax the body and mind. Test out methods like the 4-7-8 approach or diaphragmatic breathing.

Physical Relaxation: Stretching, tai chi, and yoga can all help lower tension and increase balance and flexibility.

Interests and Passtimes Read, garden, or listen to music—among other happy and relaxing pastimes.

Administration: For emotional support as well as to share your experiences and difficulties, turn to friends, family, and support groups.

Technology Supporting Diabetes Management
Numerous tools are available in modern

technology to assist with better diabetes management:

Continuous Glucose Monitors (CGMs): These devices help to keep better control by offering real-time blood sugar readings and high and low warnings.
Apps for managing diabetes on a smartphone can monitor food, exercise, blood sugar, and prescriptions. Reminds and instructional materials are other features of some apps.
Telemedicine: Getting guidance and help from medical professionals virtually can be quite easy.
Social Media Groups To find support and similar experiences with other people managing diabetes, join social media groups and internet forums.
Advice on Sustaining Long-Term Success It takes a long-term dedication and lifestyle adjustments to maintain the advantages of Dr. Barbara's treatment plan. Following are some pointers to keep success:

Clearly State Your Goals: Clearly state your goals for weight management, blood sugar control, and general health.
Keep Up to Date Follow the most recent

developments in diabetes management research and advice.

Frequent Check-Ups Plan routine checkups with your doctor to track your development and make necessary treatment plan adjustments.

Honor Significant Achievers Acknowledge and enjoy your accomplishments, no matter how modest. Confidence and drive can both increase as result.

Flexibility and Adaptability: As life happens, be ready to modify your strategy. Long-term success depends critically on flexibility and adaptation.

Case Studies Integrating Practically in Daily Life

Following are some instances of how patients have effectively included Dr. Barbara's treatment plan into their everyday lives:

James, a fifty-year-old teacher, was diagnosed with Type 2 Diabetes five years ago. He battled to regulate his weight and blood sugar. Once Dr. Barbara began her therapy, he set up a daily schedule that comprised:

Taking his prescriptions during his morning

and evening meals.
Sundays are spent cooking wholesome meals for the next week.
Every morning, before work, I spend thirty minutes walking.
Following his blood sugar levels with a CGM and a diabetes management app.
Ten minutes a night of mindfulness meditation practice to lower stress.
The result was that James lost 20 pounds in six months and his HbA1c levels fell from 8.2% to 6.5%. He has greater energy and feels more in charge of his diabetes.

Case Study 2: Laura Adjusts
Twenty years ago, 35-year-old nurse Laura received a Type 1 Diabetes diagnosis. It was difficult to manage her illness while putting in long days at work. Adopting Dr. Barbara's approach, she included the following procedures:

Insulin distribution and monitoring done precisely with a CGM and insulin pump.
Preparing meals on her days off to make sure she got wholesome, well-balanced meals when working shifts.
Short, intense workouts throughout her lunch breaks.

Taking weekly yoga lessons could help control stress.
Taking part in an internet support group for diabetes to get guidance and emotional support.
Result: Laura had less blood sugar swings and her HbA1c dropped from 7.9% to 6.8%. Though her work is challenging, she feels more balanced and less anxious.

Overcoming Typical Obstacles
In spite of their best efforts, patients could have trouble incorporating the treatment regimen into their everyday lives. This is how to get over some typical obstacles:

Time Restrictions

Barrier: Trying to fit in exercise, diet preparation, and stress management can be challenging with hectic schedules.
Solution: Set up time and give health activities top priority, even if it means dividing them into smaller, easier-to-manage chores.
Not Motivated:

Barrier: It can be difficult to keep up the drive for long-term lifestyle adjustments.

Solution: Give yourself little, doable rewards for reaching your goals. Look for help from a health coach, friends, or family.
Limited Resources:

Barrier: Buying prescription drugs, monitoring equipment, and healthful food can be quite expensive.
Solution: Check into generic drug possibilities, meal planning that is within your budget, and help programs.
The pressures of society and culture:

Barrier: Diabetes control may be at odds with cultural customs and social gatherings.
Solution: Make social event plans in advance, look for healthful, culturally appropriate substitutes, and let friends and family know what you require.
Emotional Difficulties

Barrier: Having diabetes can be hampered by stress, worry, and sadness.
Solution: Practice stress-reduction tactics, see a therapist for expert assistance, and join in encouraging social networks.
Synopsis
Creating a regimented schedule, eating a diabetes-friendly diet, getting regular

exercise, controlling stress, using technology, and getting over typical obstacles are all part of implementing Dr. Barbara's treatment plan into daily life. This chapter shows, using actual case studies and useful advice, that patients can succeed in long-term diabetes management provided they are committed and flexible. Even with diabetes, people can live healthier, more satisfying lives by being proactive and making use of the tools and assistance that are available. The benefits of better health and well-being outweigh the sometimes difficult journey.

Chapter 7: Moving Forward

Research Advancements in Diabetes

Diabetes research is an ever-evolving subject where many discoveries have the potential to completely change how we view and treat this chronic disease. The following important domains are seeing major developments:

1. Artificial Pancreas Systems: By fusing an insulin pump with a continuous glucose monitor (CGM), these systems simulate the actions of a normal pancreas to automate blood sugar control. The most recent versions lower the cost of diabetes care and enhance blood sugar control by using sophisticated algorithms to modify insulin delivery in real time.

Researchers are creating insulin formulations that will activate automatically when blood sugar levels rise. With less shots and a reduced chance of hypoglycemia, these smart insulins seek to offer better control.

2. Beta-Cell Replacement: Researchers studying stem cells are progressing in manufacturing beta cells that patients can get as transplants. By getting the body back to producing insulin, this method may offer a long-term cure for Type 1 Diabetes.

3. Gene Editing: Genetic abnormalities causing diabetes are being investigated using methods such as CRISPR-Cas9. With monogenic forms of diabetes in particular, this may result in therapies that target the underlying cause of the condition.

4. Gut microbiome research: Immune system and metabolism are greatly influenced by the gut microbiome. New directions for the treatment of diabetes are being explored by research into how altering the gut flora can increase insulin sensitivity and lower inflammation.

5. Non-Invasive Glucose Monitoring: The creation of wearable devices that test glucose via the skin or contact lenses that record glucose levels in tears is being facilitated by developments in sensor technology. These advancements try to simplify and increase accessibility of

glucose monitoring.

Technology's Place in Diabetes Care

Through tools that improve monitoring, increase medication adherence, and provide individualized assistance, technology is revolutionizing diabetes care. Among the ways technology is changing things are as follows:

1. Patient tracking of blood sugar levels, prescriptions, food, and exercise is made possible via mobile health apps. Numerous apps also include reminders, educational materials, and data-sharing features with medical professionals.

2. Virtual consultations in telemedicine let patients get support and medical guidance from the comfort of their homes. Those with restricted mobility or living in distant locations will especially benefit from this.

3. Wearables: To assist patients maintain their general health and keep active, wearables such as smartwatches and fitness trackers track heart rate, physical activity, and other health indicators.

Artificial intelligence, or AI, is the ability of computers to examine vast volumes of data from insulin pumps, CGMs, and other devices in order to offer individualized insights and treatment suggestions. AI is also being applied to forecast changes in blood sugar and recommend preventative actions.

4. Data Integration: Platforms that combine data from several sources (CGMs, insulin pumps, fitness trackers, etc.) offer a complete picture of a patient's health, facilitating better coordinated care and better-informed decision-making.

5. Personalized Therapy and Medicine
Personalized medicine—treatment strategies catered to a person's genetic makeup, way of life, and preferences—will increasingly dominate diabetes therapy in the future. This method, which attends to the particular requirements of every patient, promises to enhance results. Important parts of customized diabetic treatment consist of:

6. Genetic Testing: Customizing treatments is made possible by identifying genetic

differences that impact diabetes risk and treatment response. For instance, owing to their genetic composition, some individuals might gain more from particular drugs.

7. Lifestyle Factors: Diet, level of exercise, stress, and other lifestyle aspects are all included in customized treatment plans. All facets of health are guaranteed to be covered by this comprehensive strategy.

8. Behavioral insights: Creating more likely-to-be-adhered-to therapies requires an understanding of a patient's behavior, preferences, and motivations. Long-lasting change can be supported by methods like behavioral coaching and motivational interviewing.

9. Precision Dosing: By using individual traits and real-time data, advanced analytics can ascertain the ideal dosage of drugs, lowering the possibility of adverse effects and increasing effectiveness.

Blending Holistic Health Methodologies

Through their attention to the social, emotional, and physical components of health, holistic health methods enhance traditional diabetes therapies. These strategies can raise general well-being and strengthen results over time. Important all-encompassing techniques consist of:

1. Nutrition: Mindful eating, balanced nutrition, and whole foods emphasize can help with blood sugar control and general health, even beyond tracking carbs. Functional nutrition takes food sensitivities and personal metabolic requirements into account.

2. Physical Activity: Diabetes management depends critically on regular exercise. Holistic methods stress sustainable and pleasurable activities like yoga, tai chi, and leisure sports.

3. Mind-Body Practices: Deep breathing, mindfulness, and meditation can all help lower stress and enhance mental health, which in turn promotes better control of diabetes.

4. Social Support: It's easier to follow treatment regimens and make good decisions when one has a network of friends,

family, and peers who can offer both practical help and emotional support.

5. Integrative Therapies: By easing pain, lowering stress, and enhancing general health, massage therapy, chiropractic care, and acupuncture can enhance traditional therapies.

Patient Education and Rights

The key to good diabetic care is patient empowerment through knowledge and self-management abilities. Better able to control their illness and make wise decisions is a proactive and knowledgeable patient. Important components of patient empowerment consist on:

1. Diabetes Education Programs: Well designed programs offer thorough instruction on all aspects of diabetes care, including food, exercise, drugs, and monitoring. Many times, these courses incorporate individualized mentoring and practical instruction.

2. Self-Management Resources: Patients who have access to resources and tools like

food diaries, exercise trackers, and blood glucose meters are better able to track their progress and make wise decisions.

Online forums and support groups provide a forum for exchanging advice, experiences, and words of encouragement. Peer support can give drive and lessen feelings of loneliness.

Encouragement of patients to speak up for themselves inside the medical system can result in better treatment and results. This covers making decisions, getting second viewpoints, and posing questions.

Healthcare Providers' Changing Role

The changing diabetes management scene heavily depends on healthcare professionals. Their responsibilities are growing to include as the field develops to include:

1. Coordinating individualized treatment regimens that combine holistic, lifestyle, and medical components is a growing responsibility of providers. This calls for cooperation amongst a diverse group.

2. Data-Driven Decision Making: By using information from several sources, healthcare professionals can decide more wisely what interventions and changes to treatments to do. This covers deciphering huge data sets with AI and analytics techniques.

3. Patient Education and Support: By acting as teachers and coaches, providers enable patients to take charge of their health and gain understanding of their illness. This calls both follow-up and constant contact.

4. Using New technology: Keeping current with and integrating new technology into practice can improve patient care. New technology, apps, and therapies must be known to providers.

5. Research and Innovation: A large number of medical professionals participate in clinical research and innovation, which advances novel procedures and therapies. Patients will thus be guaranteed access to the most recent developments in treatment.

Public Health and Policy Future Directions

Diabetes management will be shaped in large part by public health policies and programs. Important topics for future attention consist of:

1. Access to Care: It is imperative that everyone have access to reasonably priced, excellent diabetic care. This covers raising the availability of diabetes education programs, cutting down on prescription expenses, and broadening insurance coverage.

2. Prevention Programs: Early detection, education, and lifestyle changes targeted at preventing diabetes can lower the prevalence of the condition. Especially crucial are programs aimed at high-risk groups.

3. Research Funding: Developing new technologies, learning about disease mechanisms, and finding new therapies all depend on ongoing funding for diabetes research.

4. Health Equity: By emphasizing socioeconomic determinants of health, such income, education, and access to healthy foods, underprivileged populations can have better diabetes results.

5. Policy Advocacy: Systemic improvements benefited by persons with diabetes can be brought about by advocacy initiatives aiming at influencing public policy. This involves arguing for increased financing for healthcare, better rules governing diabetic supplies and drugs, and encouraging policies at work.

Synopsis

With the fast developments in research, technology, individualized treatment, and holistic health strategies, the future of diabetes care seems bright. Patients can have better results and a higher quality of life by including these developments into their daily lives. Shaping this future will need empowering patients through knowledge and assistance, as well as changing healthcare professional roles and public health programs. With ongoing advances in our knowledge of and ability to treat

72

diabetes, millions of people worldwide should eventually be able to live healthier lives because managing this illness will be easier and more efficient.

Conclusion

Finally, a New Day in Diabetes Care and Treatment
"DR. BARBARA CURE FOR DIABETES" is a groundbreaking book that goes beyond standard diabetes care. It provides cutting-edge research, unique treatment procedures, and a holistic approach to treating one of today's most common chronic diseases. In addition to carefully outlining the clinical procedures and scientific discoveries that underpin her approach throughout the book, Dr. Barbara also includes patient success stories and personal accounts that demonstrate the revolutionary power of her techniques.

Converging Clinical Applications with Scientific Advancements
Deep knowledge of the pathophysiology of diabetes is at the core of Dr. Barbara's treatment. The book breaks apart the many processes underlying beta-cell failure, insulin resistance, and the intricate interactions between heredity and environment that lead to the beginning and development of diabetes. Through the

solving of these biological puzzles, Dr. Barbara prepares the audience for the introduction of a number of cutting-edge treatment plans that seek to not only control but even to reverse diabetes.

Including state-of-the-art biotechnological developments is one of Dr. Barbara's pillars of her approach. She explores the possibilities of gene treatment, which is changing particular genes to increase insulin synthesis or lower insulin resistance. With the promise to address the underlying molecular cause of diabetes, this groundbreaking method offers hope for a long-term treatment. The fascinating field of stem cell therapy is also covered in the book. Here, injured pancreatic tissue is rebuilt using stem cells obtained from the patient, therefore restoring its capacity to manufacture insulin on its own.

A further important feature of the book is its thorough analysis of individualized medicine. Understanding that diabetes presents differently in every person, Dr. Barbara promotes a customized approach to diabetes management. Using cutting edge diagnostic instruments and biomarkers, she suggests a tailored course of therapy that fits the patient's lifestyle, genetic makeup, and particular metabolic issues. More efficient and long-lasting diabetic care is made possible by this precision medicine approach, which also reduces side effects.

Holistic and Integrative Methodologies Beyond the fields of individualized medicine and technologies, "DR. BARBARA CURE FOR DIABETES" highlights the need of lifestyle modifications and integrative health techniques. Dr. Barbara stresses that as essential elements of diabetic care, diet, exercise, and stress management are crucial. Her recommendations for a balanced macronutrient distribution, low-glycemic index meals, and the addition of antioxidant- and anti-inflammatory-rich foods are supported by scientific research.

Besides, the book emphasizes the therapeutic possibilities of complementary and alternative therapies. Dr. Barbara looks at the ways that age-old therapies like acupuncture, herbal medicine, and mindfulness meditation might help control blood sugar levels and improve general health. These integrative methods are offered to supplement traditional medical therapies rather than to replace them, therefore forming a thorough and multidimensional plan to fight diabetes.

Viewpoints and Success Stories from Patients

Dr. Barbara's techniques are brought to life by moving patient stories woven across clinical observations and scientific discussion. These success tales of people who have used her method to effectively reverse their diabetes provide those battling the illness hope and concrete proof of its effectiveness. From those with recently diagnosed diabetes to long-term sufferers, the book's varied case studies show that there is always time to start the road to recovery.

By use of these stories, Dr. Barbara also tackles the psychological and emotional components of having diabetes. She stresses the value of empowering, educating, and actively participating patients in their own care. Patients who feel more agency and self-efficacy are more able to follow their treatment plans and adopt long-lasting lifestyle modifications.

More General Social Consequences

Beyond the health of each person, Dr. Barbara's treatment has ramifications for society and the economy. A worldwide epidemic, diabetes places heavy demands on economies and healthcare systems everywhere. The book makes the case that implementing Dr. Barbara's creative and all-encompassing strategy could result in significant savings in hospital stays, healthcare expenses, and complications associated to diabetes. This change will not only raise personal quality of life but also lessen the financial burden on the infrastructure supporting public health.

Dr. Barbara also demands that public health laws and healthcare delivery systems be changed structurally. She is in favor of more money going into diabetes research, more people having access to cutting-edge therapies, and lifestyle medicine being included into routine treatment plans. Her goal goes beyond health justice and the social determinants of health to include a world in which everyone, regardless of financial situation, can avoid and treat diabetes.

Perspective on the Future
Looking ahead, "DR. BARBARA CURE FOR DIABETES" provides a bold road plan for revolutionizing diabetes care. It is possible to treat diabetes not only manage it by combining technologies, individualized

medicine, and integrative health approaches. In her ideal future, Dr. Barbara sees genetic and stem cell treatments restoring normal pancreatic function, early detection and intervention stopping the disease in its tracks, and long-term health maintenance achieved by holistic lifestyle changes.

In improving diabetic care, the book also predicts how artificial intelligence and digital health technology will develop. Real-time modifications and preemptive interventions made possible by wearable devices, continuous glucose monitoring, and AI-driven analytics may completely change how patients and healthcare professionals monitor and manage the condition.

Conclusions
More than simply a medical book, "DR. BARBARA CURE FOR DIABETES" offers millions of people worldwide hope. The all-encompassing and holistic method of treatment that Dr. Barbara presents offers a paradigm change in our knowledge of, approach to managing, and ultimate goal to cure diabetes. Making a strong argument for the viability of a diabetes-free future, she closes the gap between cutting-edge research and practical application by fusing scientific rigor with compassionate care.

This book is, in the end, a monument to the human spirit's tenacity, the ability of creativity, and the possibility of revolutionary transformation in the healthcare industry. It extends a welcome to patients, medical professionals, academics, and decision-makers to participate in the joint battle against diabetes. With the dawn of this new century, "DR. BARBARA CURE FOR DIABETES" acts as a beacon, showing the way to a healthy, diabetes-free society.

This summary of Dr. Barbara's work highlights the clinical, scientific, and human aspects of her strategy for treating diabetes. With an eye on motivating readers to work together to address this worldwide health issue, it considers the wider ramifications and future opportunities.

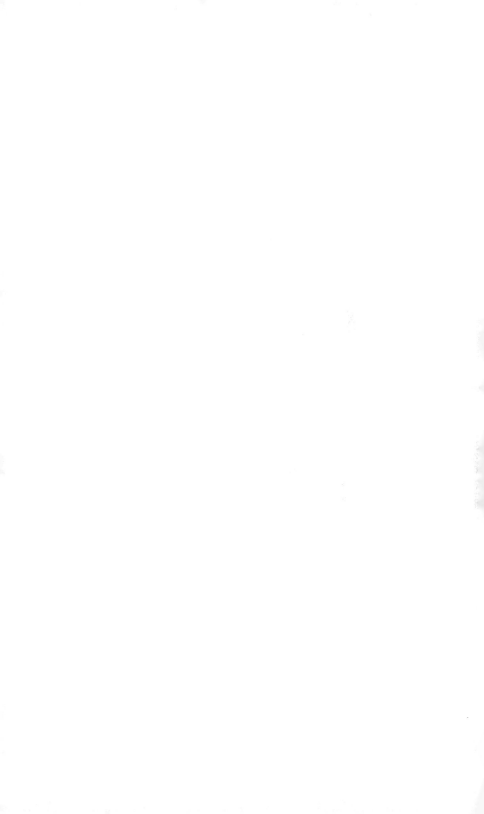

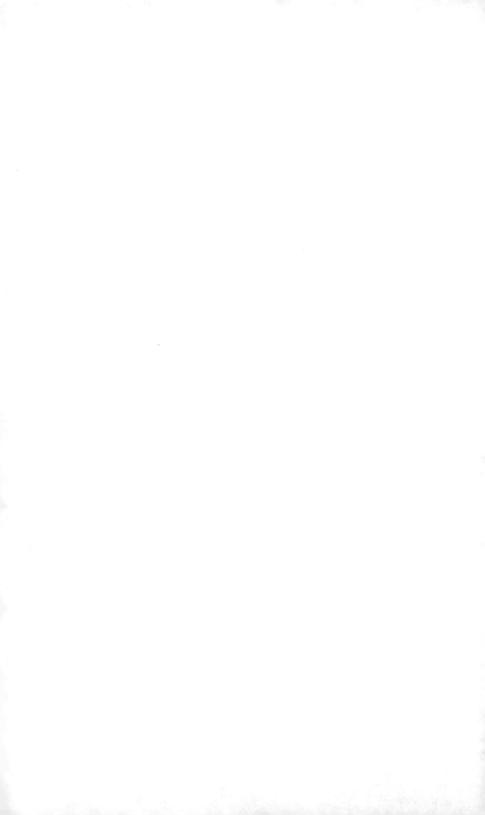

Made in the USA
Las Vegas, NV
23 August 2024

b32af3af-18ea-40ba-82bb-a50343e3089cR01